An exciting adventure that illustrates the importance of plant-based nutrition to children.

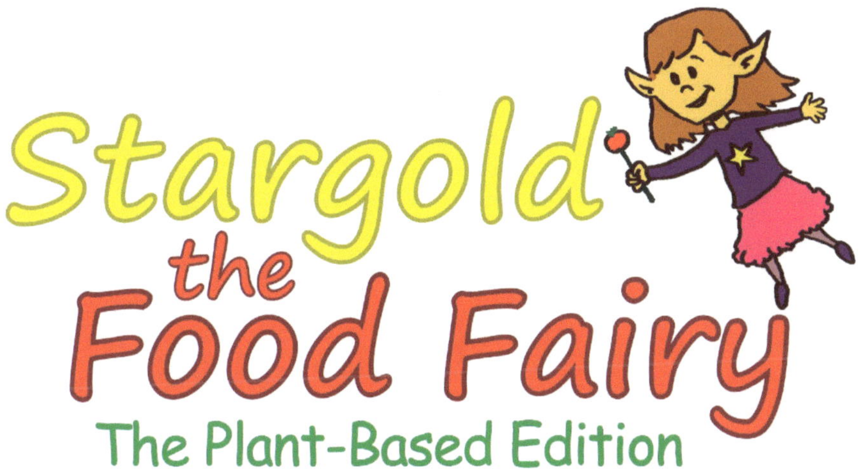

written by
Claudia Lemay, RD

with the collaboration of
Vesanto Melina, MS, RD

illustrations by
Chris Hamilton

"Good foods build the brain; good books expand it."

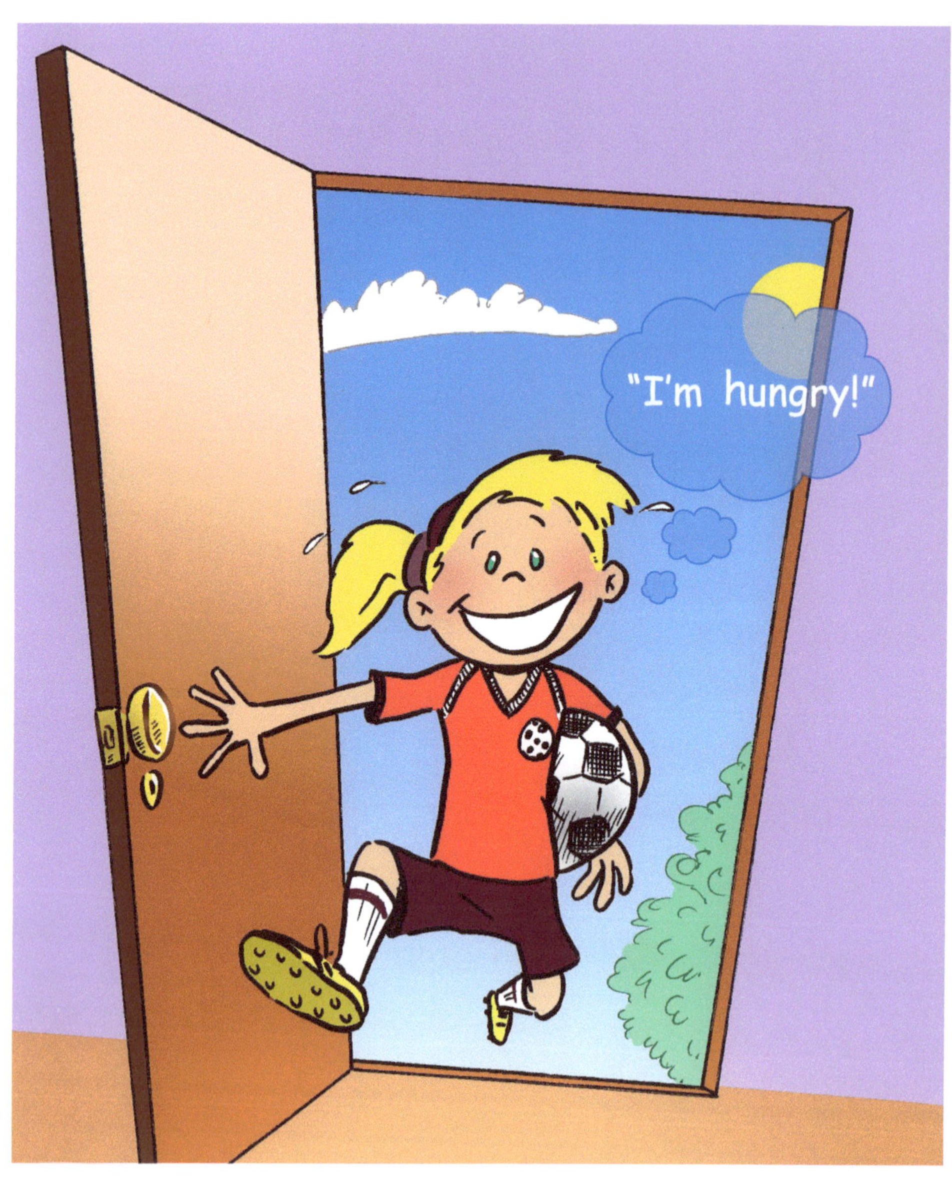

The other day, when Lucie came home from soccer practice, she was super-duper extra hungry. She ran through the kitchen door and rushed to the pantry, looking for candy.

"Oh hello, Lucie," said her mother. "I was just putting dinner on the table. It's a nice tofu scramble full of vegetables!"

Lucie looked at the food on her plate.

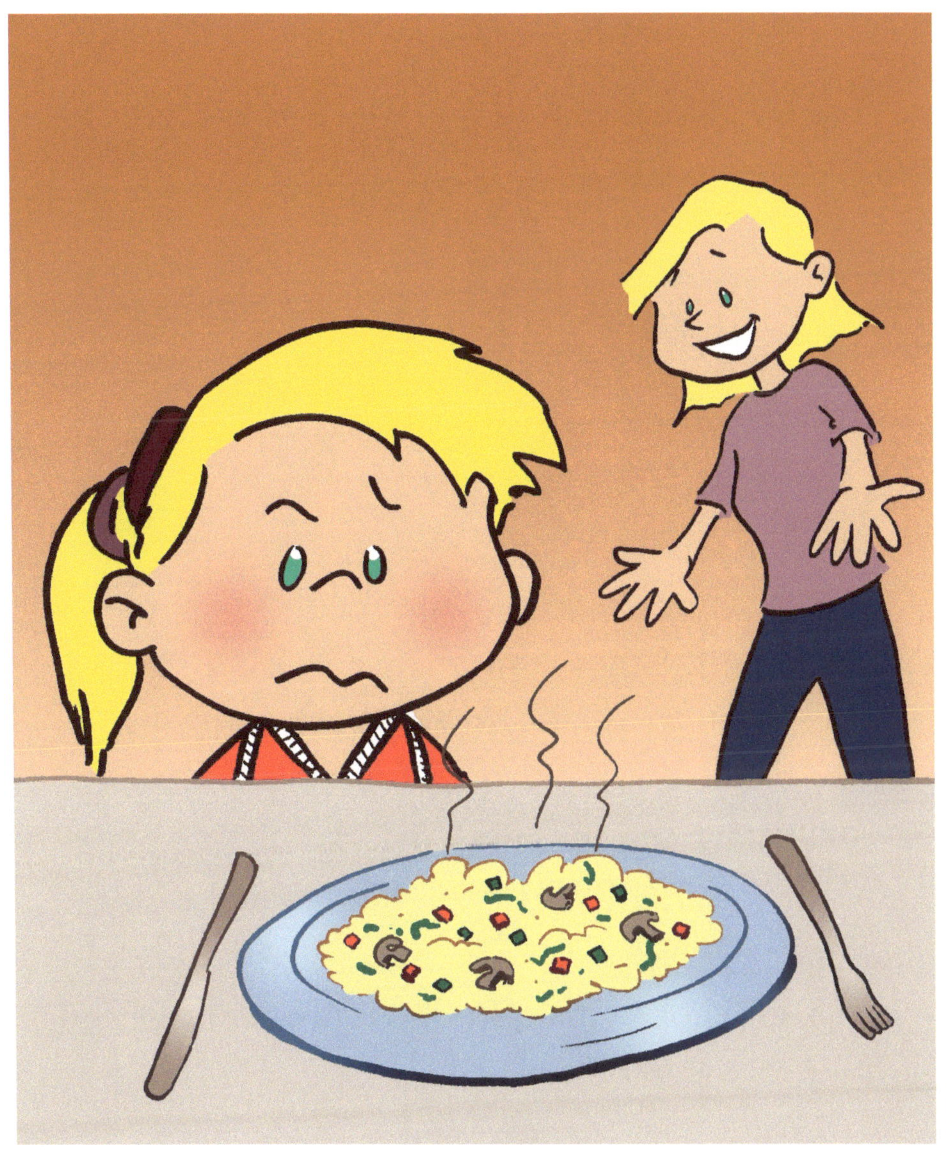

"I don't want that," she said. "I want vegan marshmallow stew with cotton candy instead!"

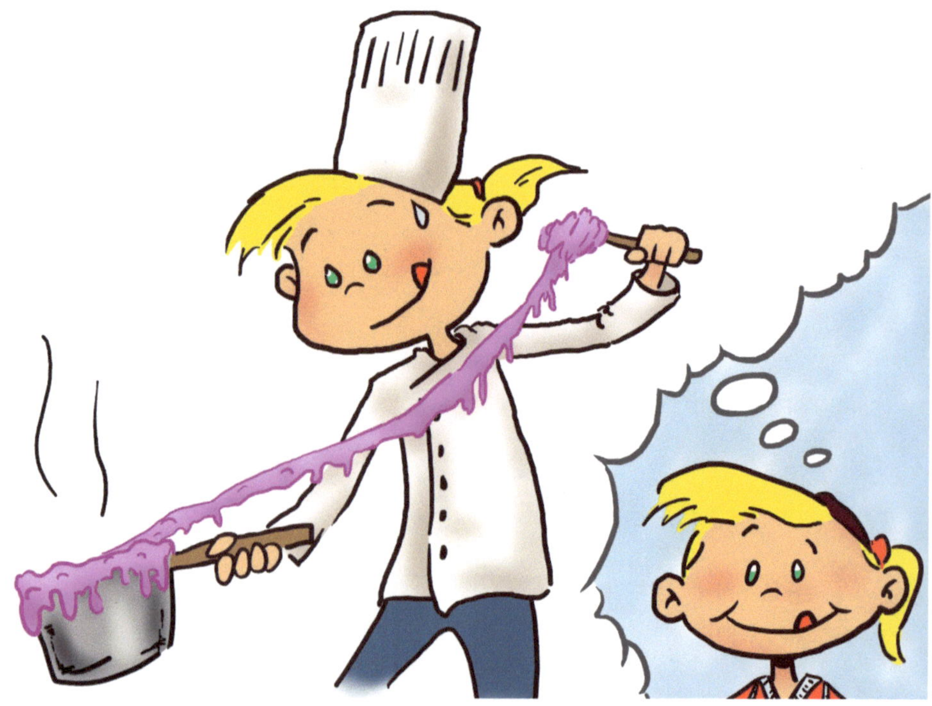

Her mother laughed. "Absolutely not, sweetie. As the parent, I choose what we eat, where we eat and when we eat it. Now go wash your hands, please."

"That's not fair," said Lucie, scrubbing her hands at the sink. "Why don't I get to make any choices?"

"Your choices are whether you eat or not and how much you eat."

"I want to eat candy," yelled Lucie.

"But that's not what I made, sweetie," insisted her mother.

"Okay, I am going to eat in my room then," she answered, secretly planning to throw it out the window to the neighbour's dog, who didn't seem fussy at all.

"How am I supposed to hear about your day then? We eat together as a family every day," replied her mother in her 'Mom Voice'.

Lucie got super angry. She got so angry, that she ran to her room, slammed the door, and stood there, sulking. She was hungry, but she did not want to eat that gross scramble! Her belly rumbled, and that's when she heard a soft 'swoosh'...

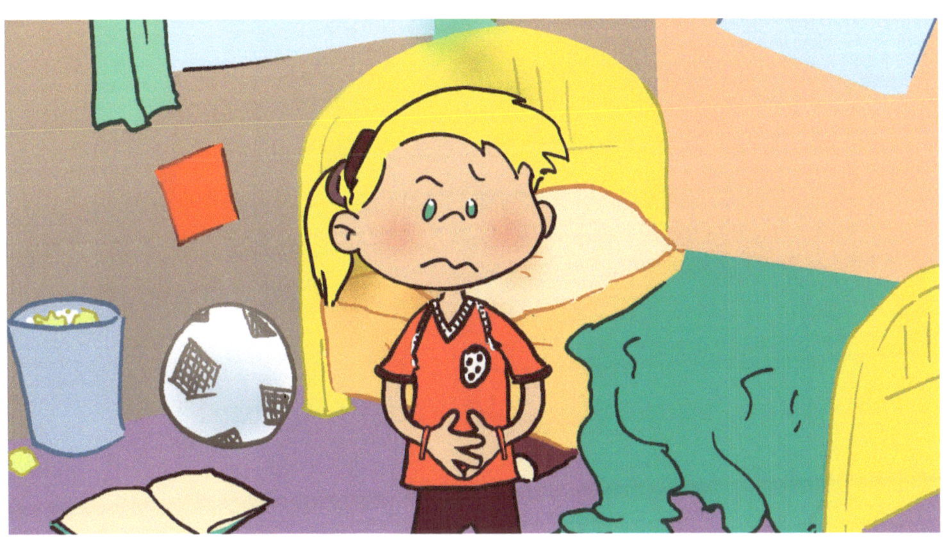

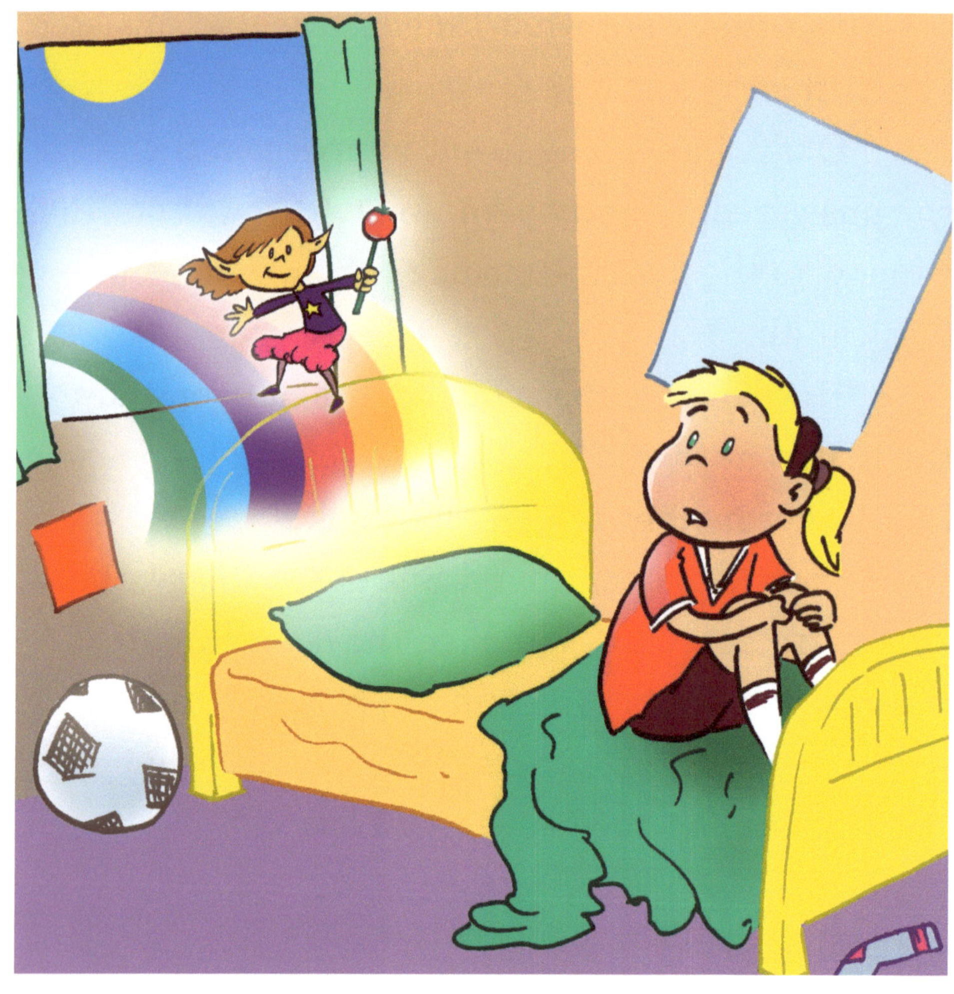

Through the window, a small creature with pointy ears had flown in, riding on a sparkling rainbow.

"Hello, Lucie," said the pointy-eared creature.

"Uh, hello," said Lucie. "Who are you?"

"My name is Stargold and I am the Food Fairy."

"What! A Food Fairy?" asked Lucie.

"I may not be as popular as my cousin, the Tooth Fairy, but my job is just as important. I help children all over the world grow strong and healthy! I want to show you Growland. Do you want to come?"

"Sure, but where did you say we are going?" asked Lucie, still hoping she might get candy.

"Growland! It's a magical place!"

"Magical? Cool! Let's go!"

Stargold took Lucie's hand and they flew out the window.

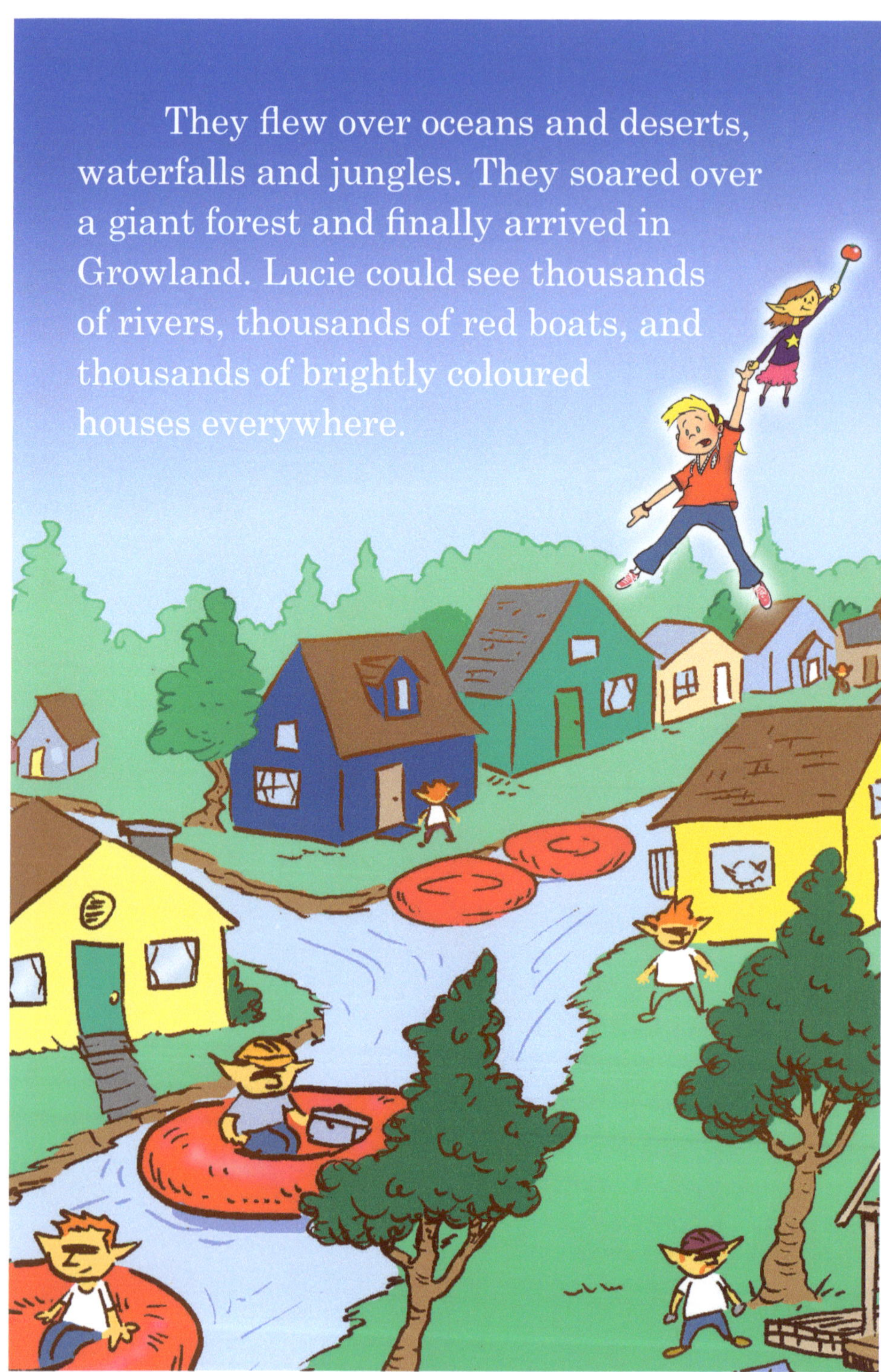

They flew over oceans and deserts,
waterfalls and jungles. They soared over
a giant forest and finally arrived in
Growland. Lucie could see thousands
of rivers, thousands of red boats, and
thousands of brightly coloured
houses everywhere.

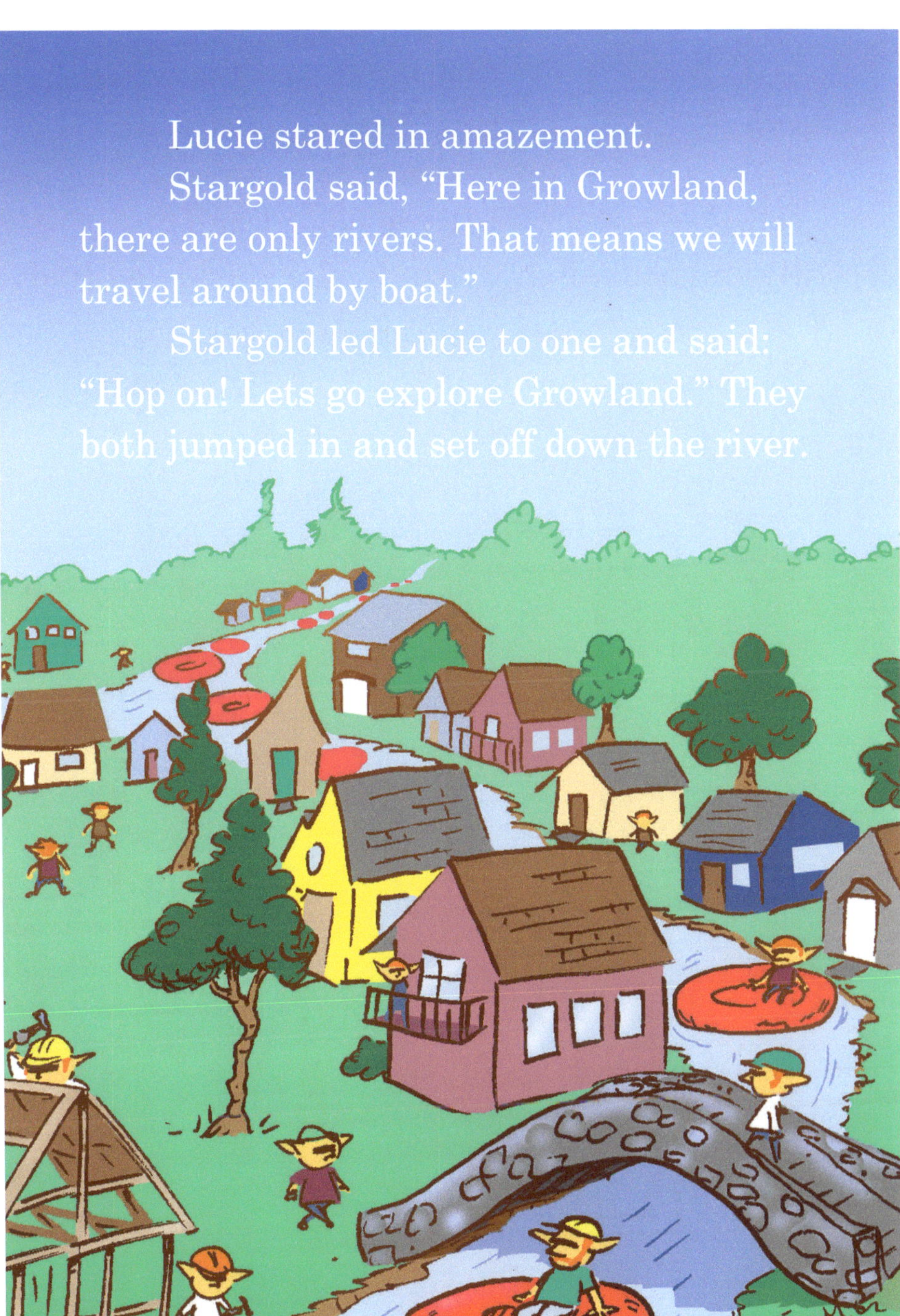

Lucie stared in amazement.

Stargold said, "Here in Growland, there are only rivers. That means we will travel around by boat."

Stargold led Lucie to one and said: "Hop on! Lets go explore Growland." They both jumped in and set off down the river.

"The Elves here build magical houses," said Stargold.

"How are they magical?" Lucie asked.

"The houses here are not real. Each one is actually the body of a person in the world you live in."

"Huh? How does that work?" asked Lucie, puzzled.

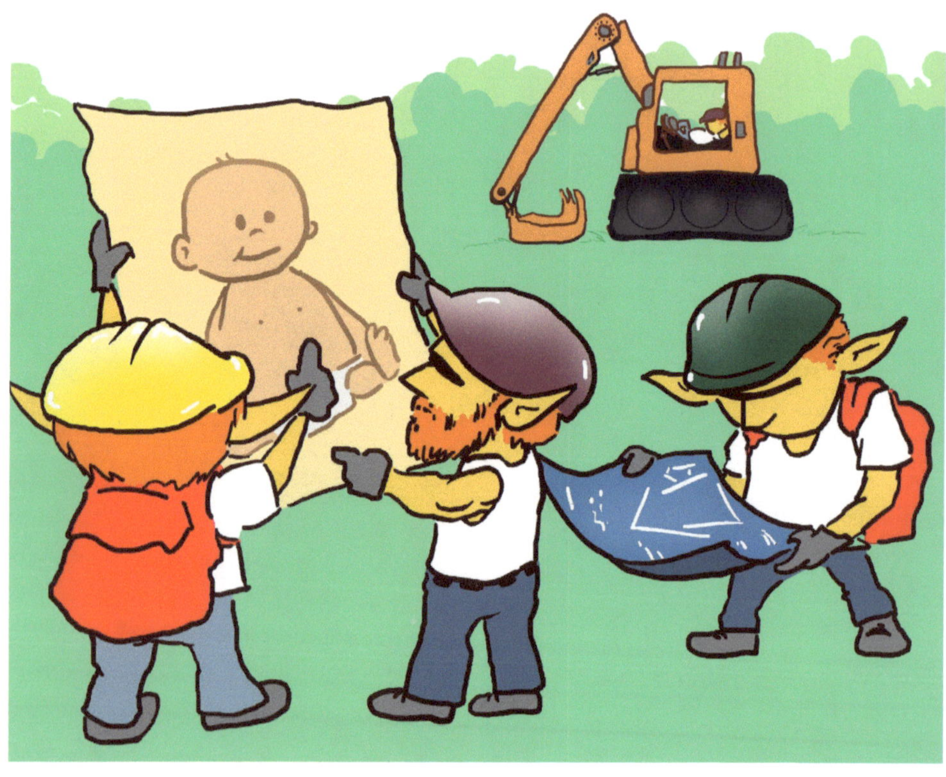

"When a mother gives birth to a baby, the Elves receive the information from the parents 'DNA' on how the baby's body is supposed to grow."

"The Elves then build the baby's body here in Growland as a house," Stargold went on, "And in your world, it grows as the baby's body."

"Wow! really?" said Lucie.

"Close your eyes, and take my hand. I have a surprise for you!"

"Oh, I love surprises," exclaimed Lucie.

Stargold brought Lucie further down the river.

"Open your eyes," she said, pointing to a cute little house. "That is YOUR house!"

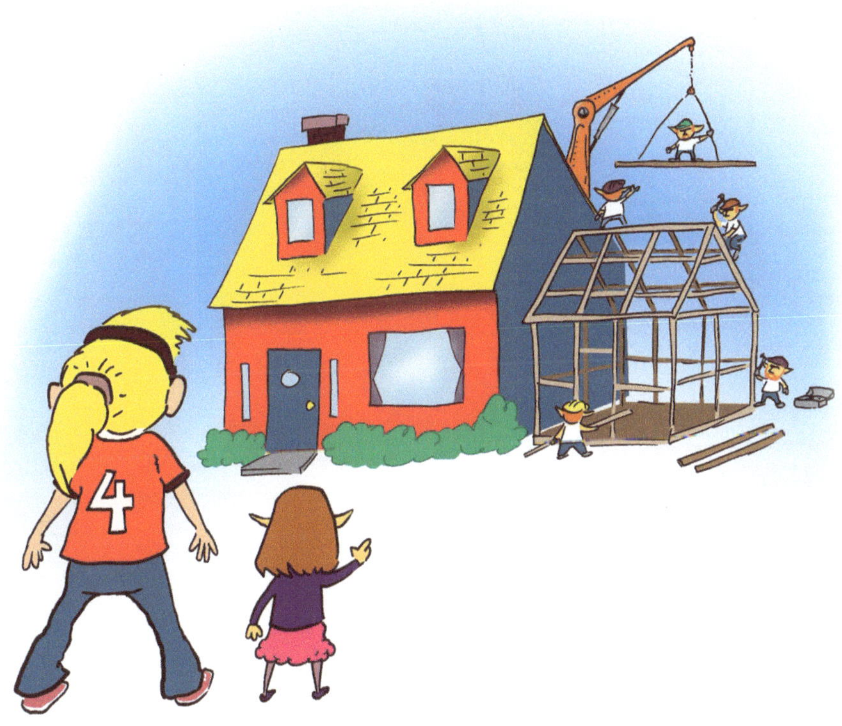

"Whoa! It looks just like me," Lucie said.

"Yes, and look how hard they are working on this one," said Stargold.

"How do the Elves build houses? " asked Lucie.

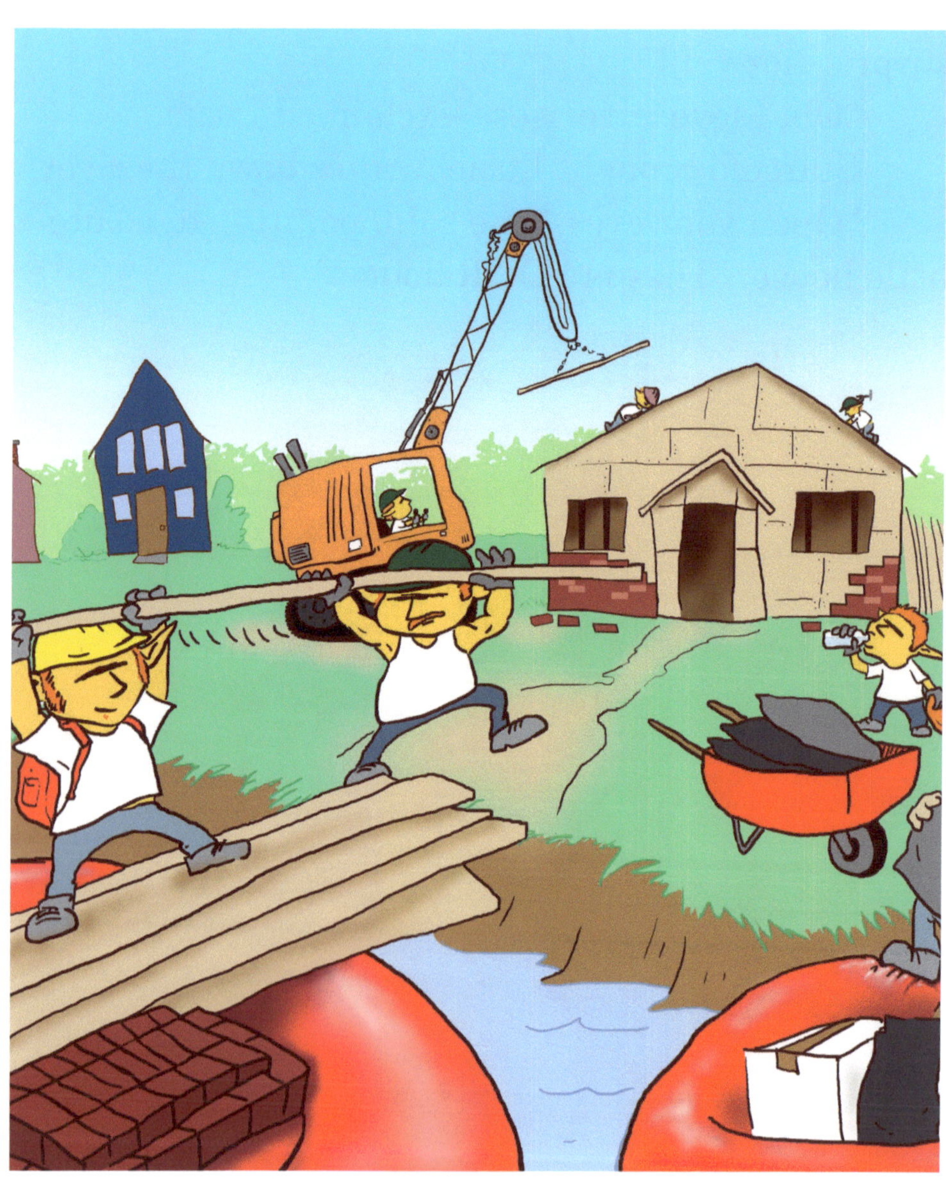

"All the necessary materials are brought in by boats to the construction site. The materials only come to the builders when that person eats something," explained Stargold.

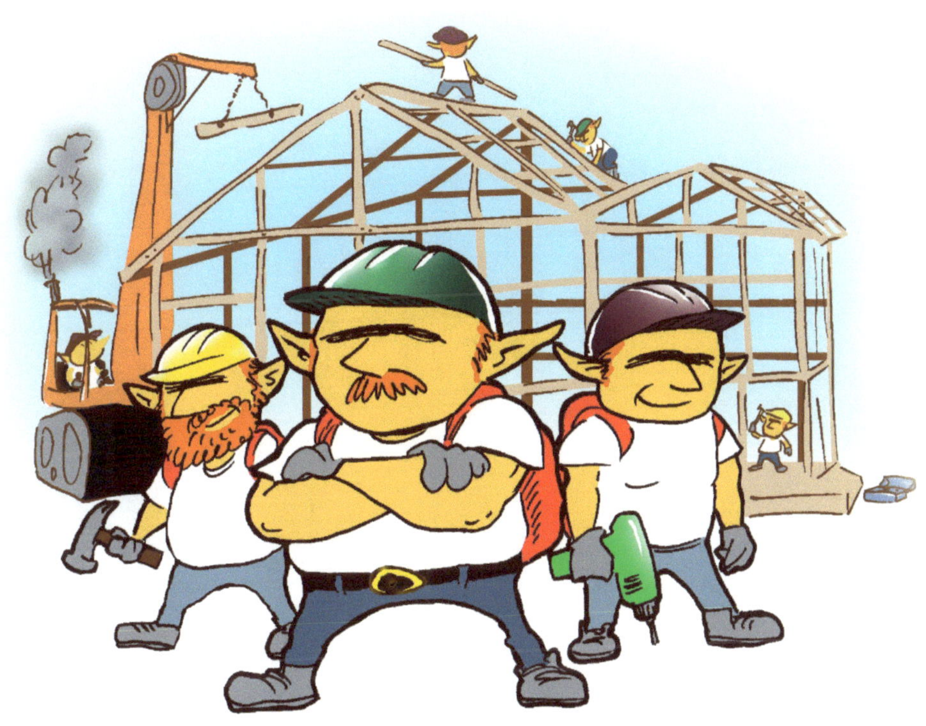

"Look! The Body Builder Elves are building the frame of an extension on your house. In your body, that would be the skeleton."

"Without the skeleton," Stargold went on,
"your body would be a big blob on the ground.
Now, watch this!" said Stargold, flicking her wand.

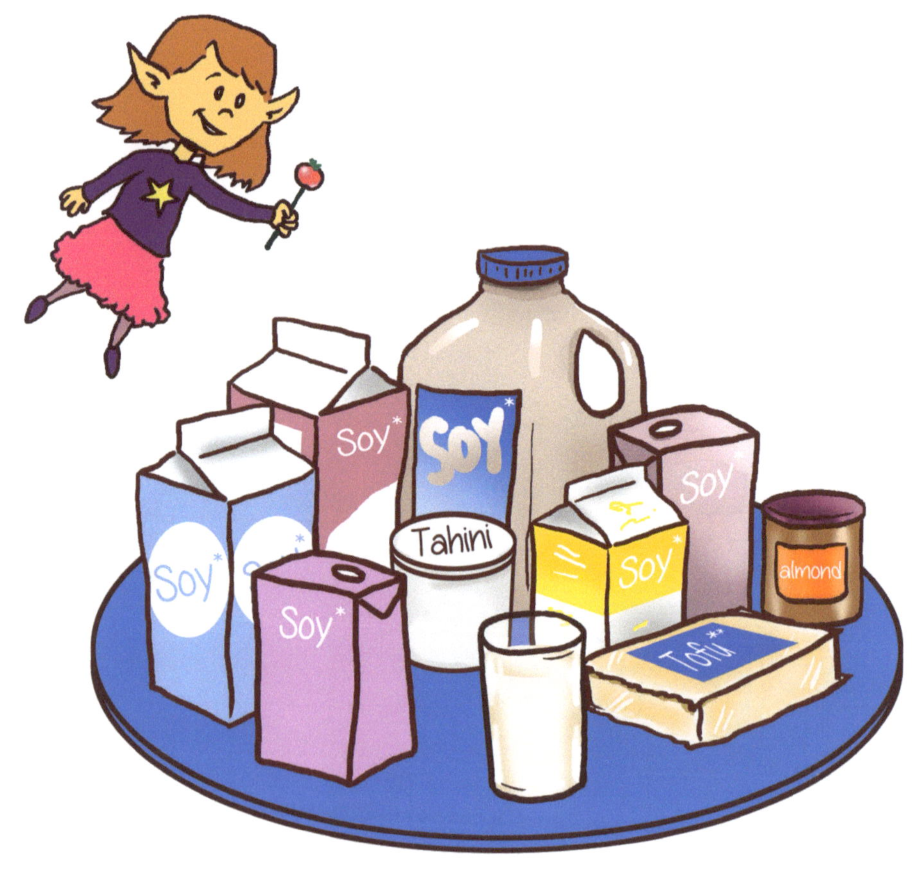

*Calcium and Vitamin D Fortified   **Calcium-set tofu*

A tray magically appeared. It was full of
different kinds of calcium-rich foods.

Stargold continued: "Calcium is the material needed to build your bones, just like wood is needed to build the frame of a house. Now drink some soy milk and watch what happens!"

Lucie took a giant gulp, and suddenly a boat came around the corner carrying large, strong boards of wood.

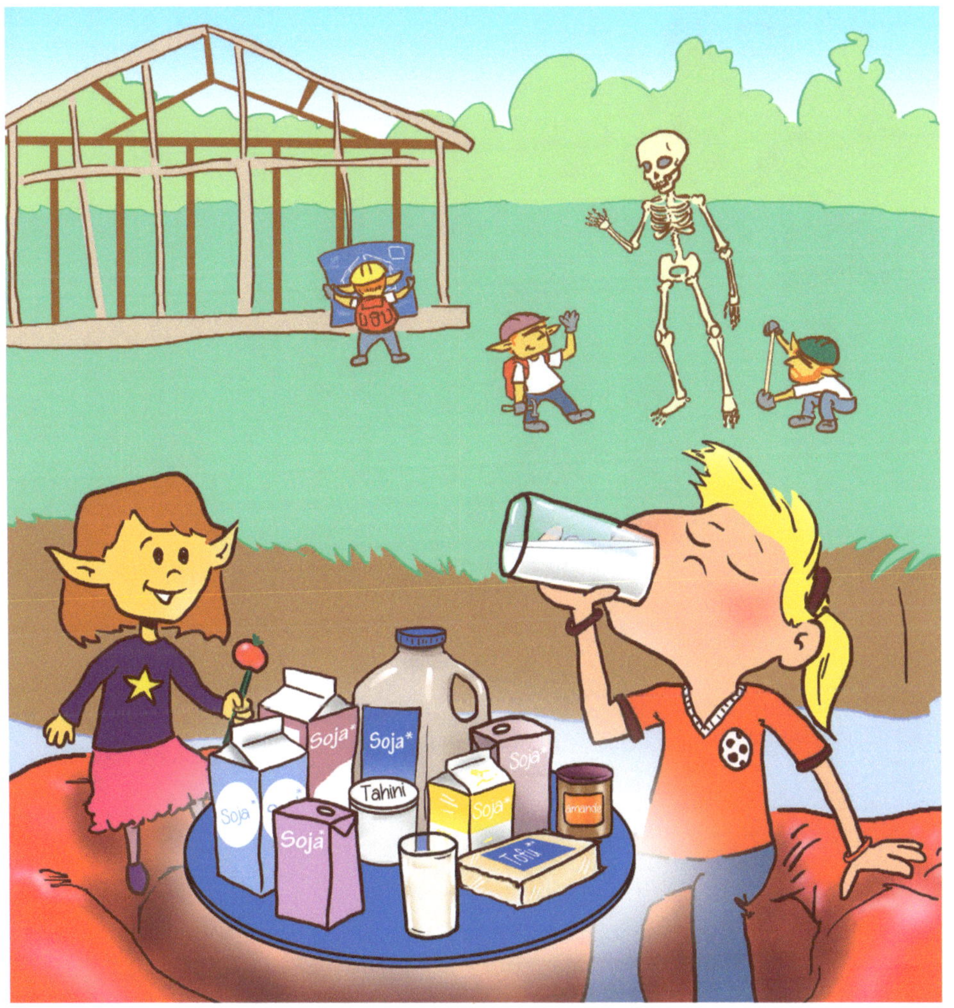

"Well done!" said Stargold. "Now the Body Builder Elves have what they need."

"Wow!" said Lucie.

"Let's see what happens next," said Stargold. She pointed to Lucie's house. "In order to make the bricks for the walls of your house, the Elves need you to eat foods that are high in protein."

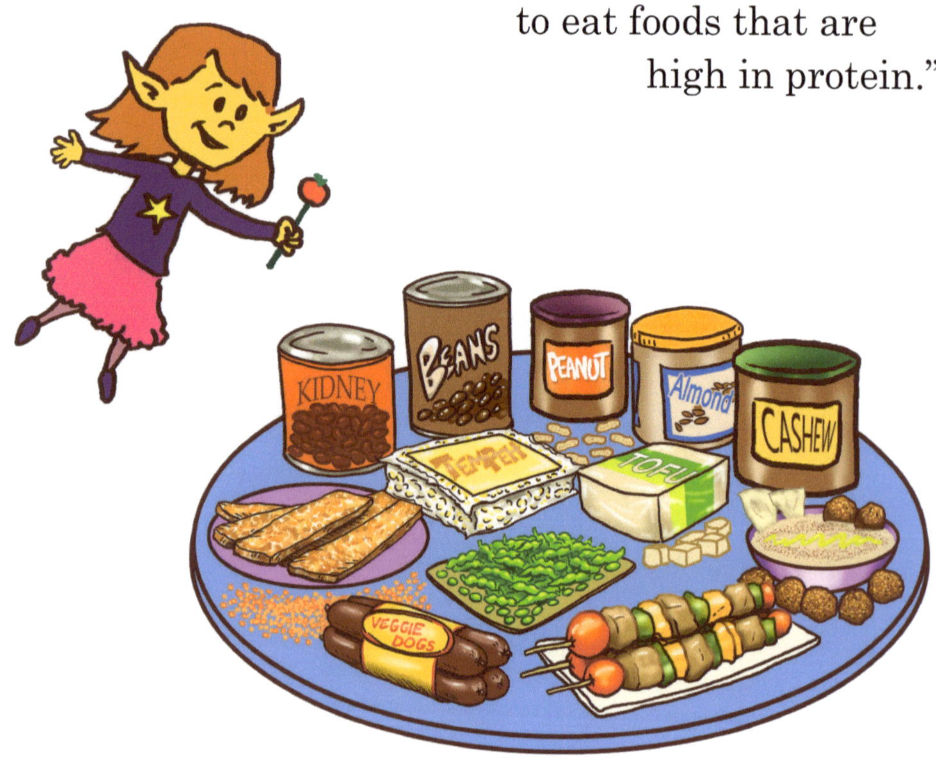

Stargold waved her wand and another tray showed up. This one was full of protein-rich foods.

"Protein is the building block of almost everything in your body – your muscles, hair, blood, skin and even your heart."

Lucie grabbed a handful of falafel patties and stuffed her cheeks.

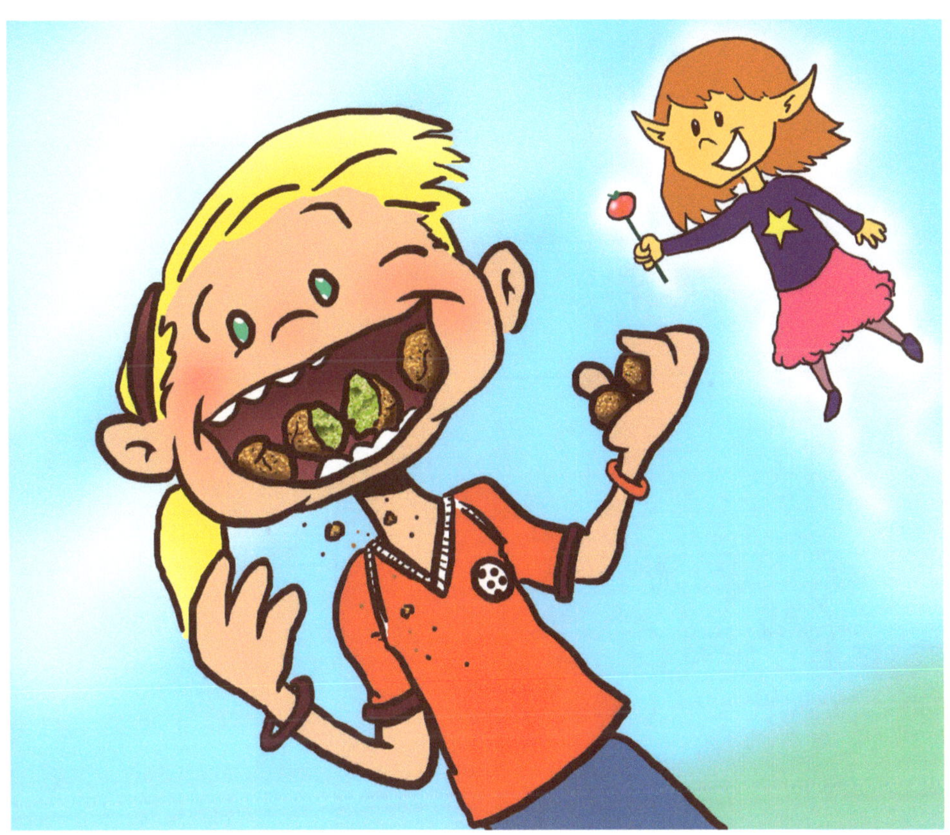

Everyone laughed. "Keep going like this, and I will have to call my aunt, the Good Manners Fairy, and start a whole other book about you, Lucie!" said Stargold, chuckling.

As Lucie chewed, a boat showed up at the dock in front of Lucie's house and the elves started unloading bricks.

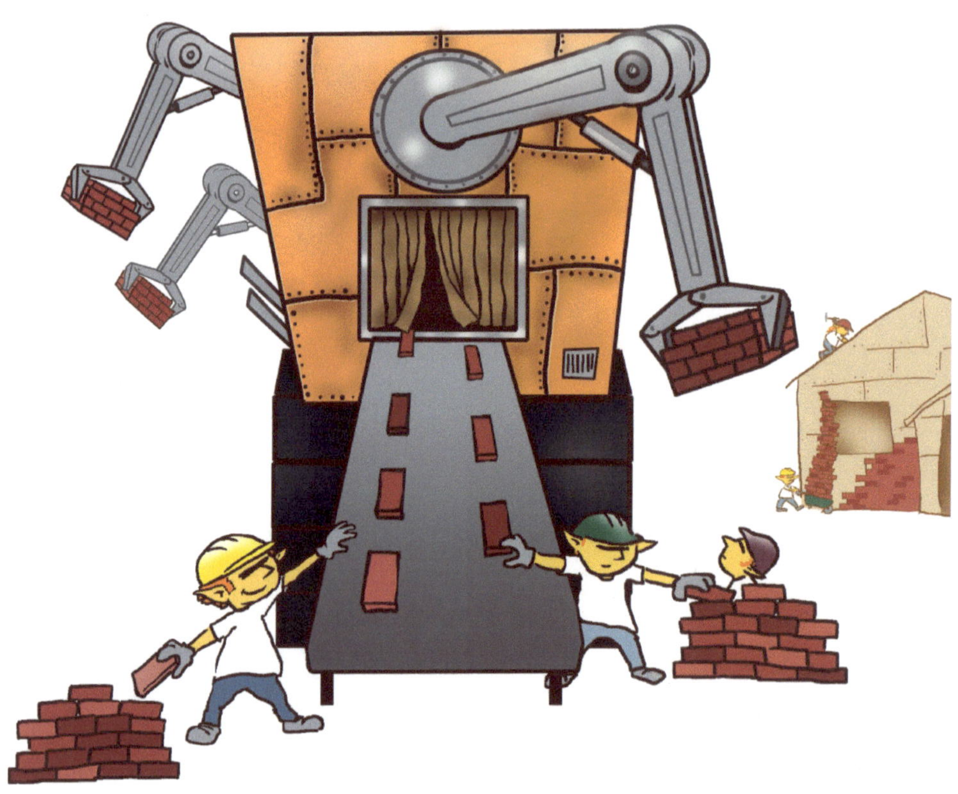

"See what just happened? Now they can build the walls of your house. With these bricks the walls will be strong, just like your muscles and your heart."

Lucie nodded, her mouth still too full of falafels to talk.

Stargold continued, "Now in order for all the parts of your body to function well together, you need your brain. The part of a house that is like your brain is the computer. You need to eat foods that are high in healthy fats so that the Geek Elves can build the computer for your house. These foods contain essential fatty acids which are the building blocks of your brain."

Stargold waved her wand and a tray with food containing healthy fats and oils appeared.

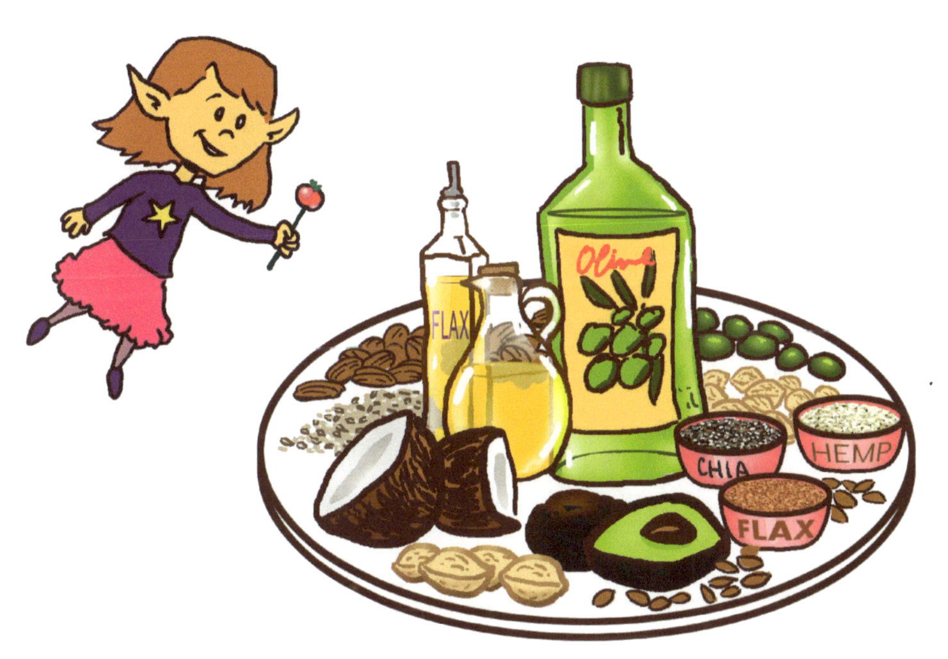

Lucie grabbed a handful of walnuts and started eating them. Stargold guided her closer to her house so she could see better.

Just then, a boat pulled up carrying computer parts that other Elves carried into Lucie's house.

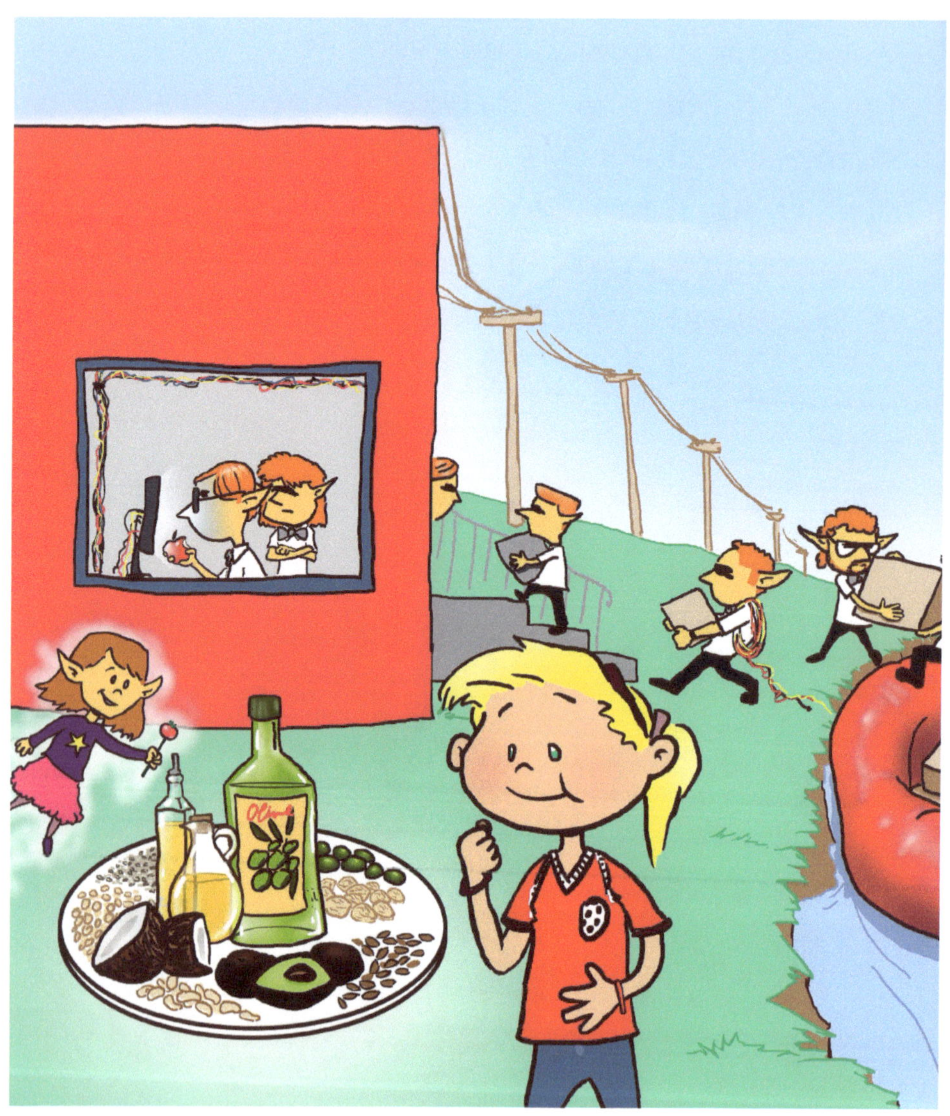

"Eating healthy oils ensures that your brain will work well. After all, building your brain is just as important as protecting it, like you do when you wear a helmet when you go biking."

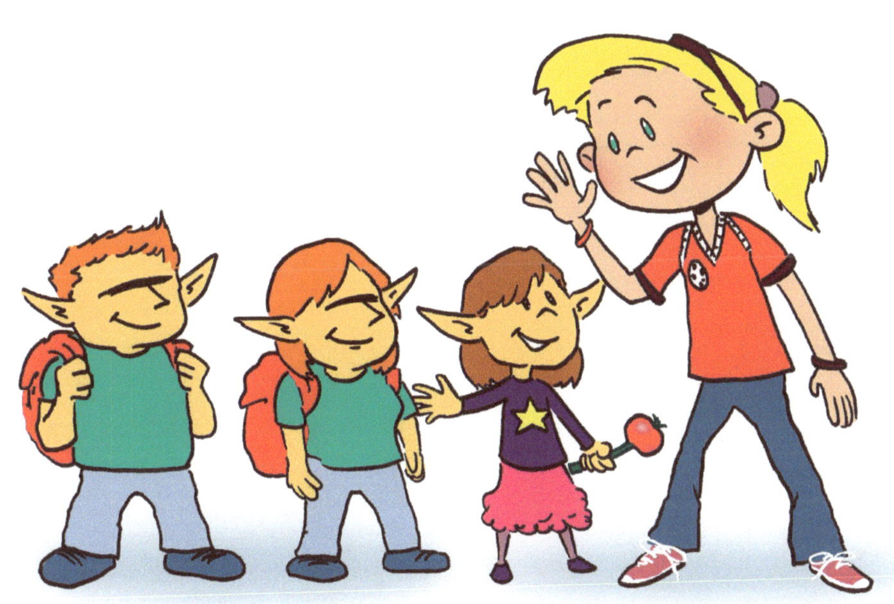

Lucie noticed two Elves walking towards them. Stargold waved them over.

"Hello! My name is Ana!" said the girl Elf.

"Hello! My name is Bolly!" said the boy Elf. "We are Junior Body Builder Elves."

"Hi, I am Lucie!" she answered.

"Could you please show Lucie what you carry in your backpacks?" asked Stargold.

"Of course," said Bolly, opening his bag for Lucie. "We carry the same things you carry in your backpack, but instead of school supplies, we bring tools."

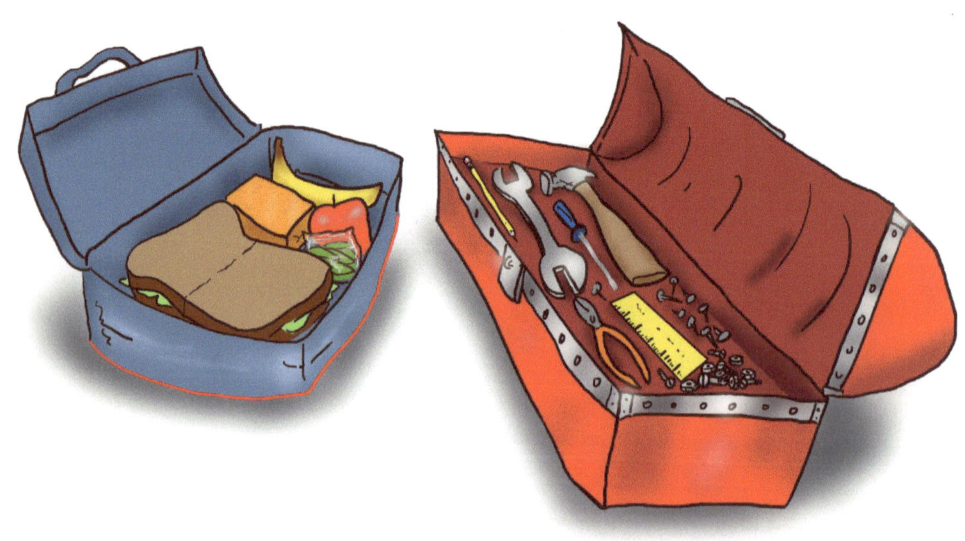

Ana continued: "When you eat whole grains, the boats bring lunch boxes for us to have the energy to build your house. Whole grains contain a lot of carbohydrates as well as vitamins and minerals. Carbohydrates give us energy, while vitamins and minerals give us tools."

"Let me show you," said Stargold.

She waved her wand and a tray with whole grain foods appeared.

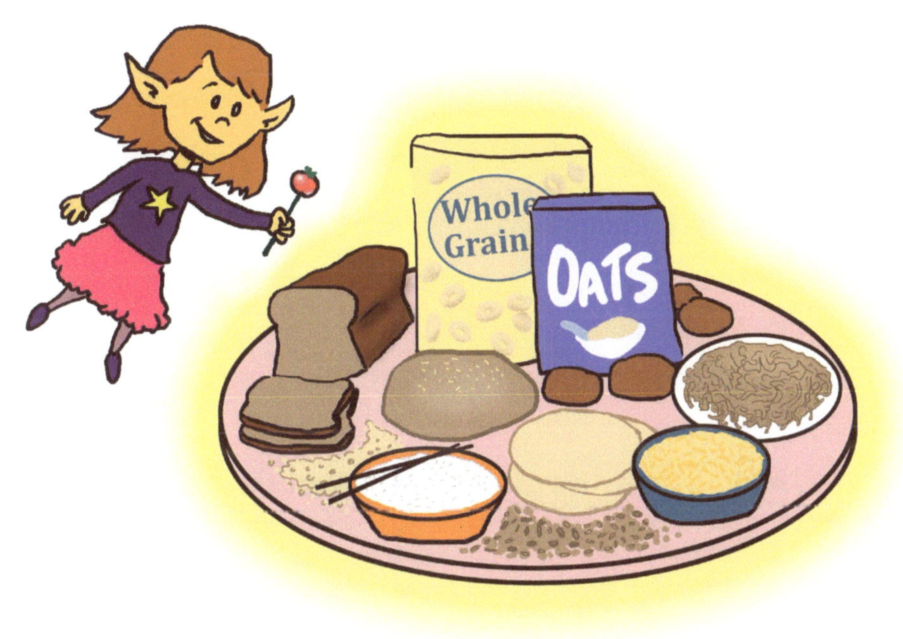

Lucie grabbed a delicious-looking whole grain roll and took a huge bite.

Right then, a boat zoomed up to the dock, and Ana and Bolly ran to fill their backpacks.

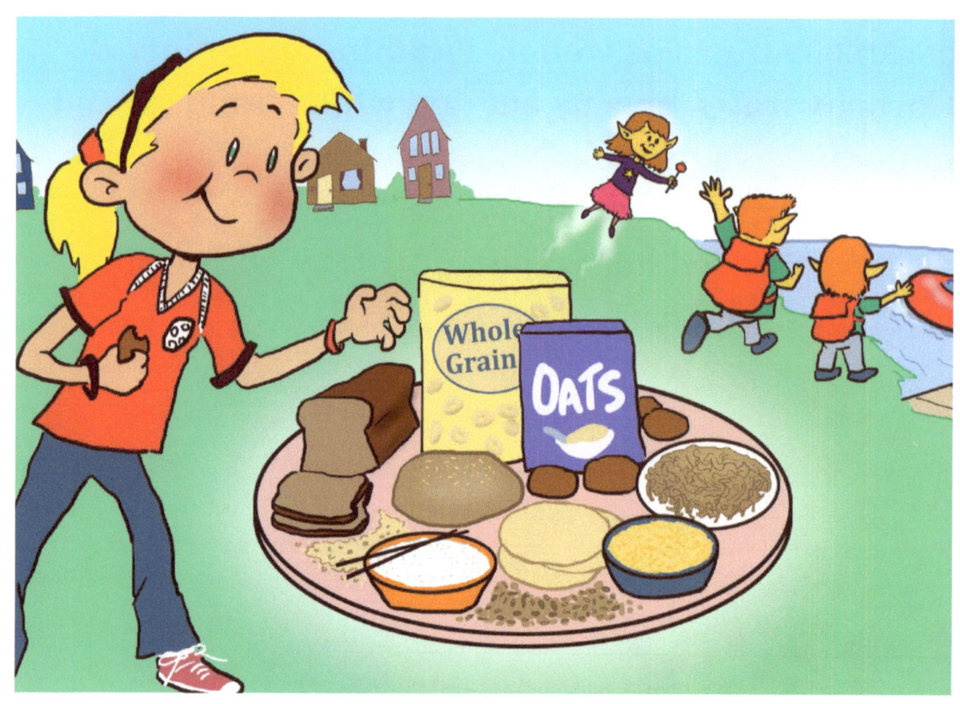

"There are other foods that contain a lot of carbohydrates: Candy, for example," said Ana, smiling.

"Yay! Stargold, make a tray of candy appear!" said Lucie.

Stargold laughed. "When you eat or drink candy, which you do when you drink soda pop, we only get lunchboxes, but zero tools! Candy doesn't have vitamins and minerals, while whole grains do. We need tools just as much as we need energy!"

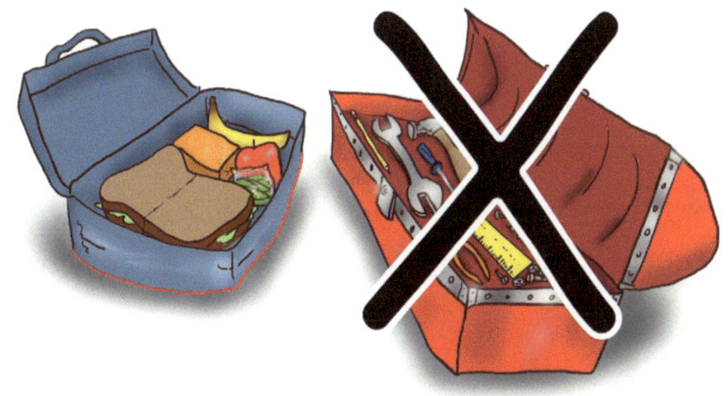

"Really?" Lucie said. "I had no idea!"

"That's why I brought you here," said Stargold. "Most kids don't know this."

"I understand now," Lucie said.

"Great. Let's go see some more."

They waved goodbye to Ana and Bolly and walked back to the river.

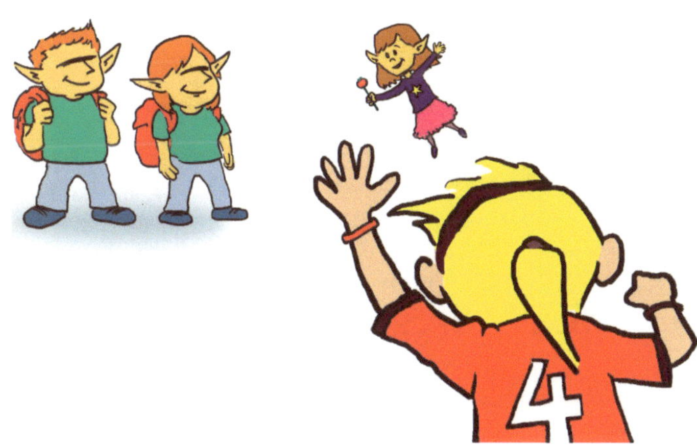

Suddenly, they heard a loud screeching noise.

Lucie looked up and saw mischievous-looking monkeys coming their way. The monkeys had climbed up onto the roof tops and were pulling shingles loose to toss at each other.

"HeeeeHeeeeeHeeee!" they said snickering.

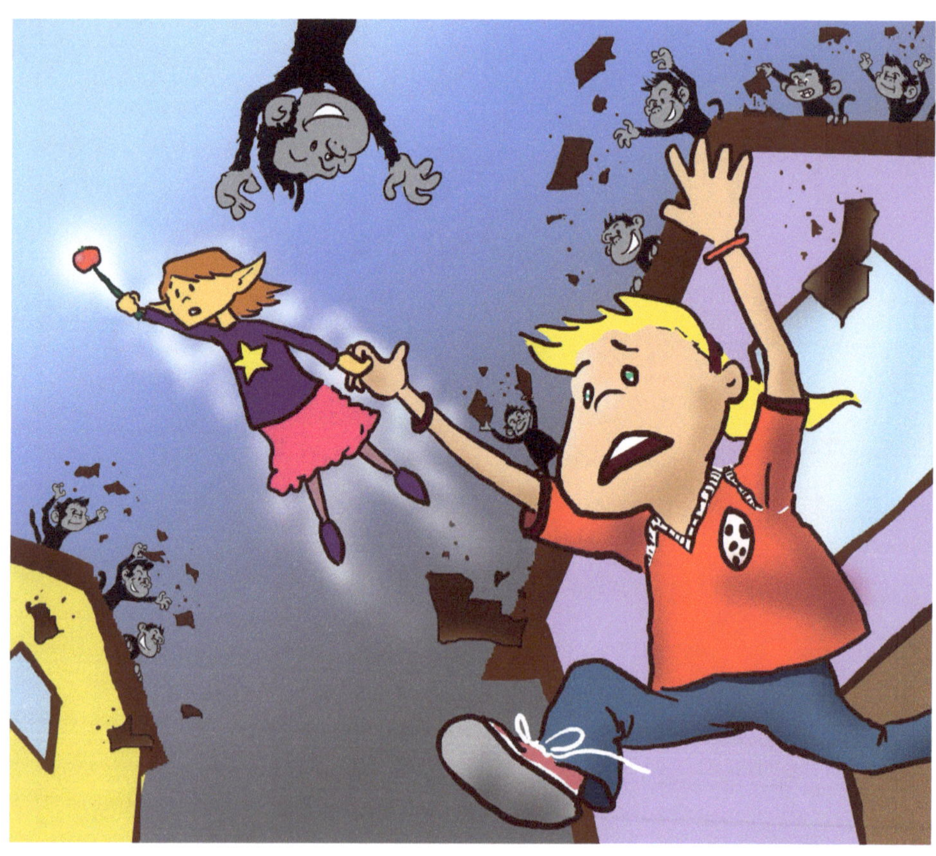

"Follow me! Quick!" Stargold yelled. "The Mayhem Monkeys are here! Let's go warn the captain!"

She grabbed Lucie's hand and they flew to the Rescue Station.

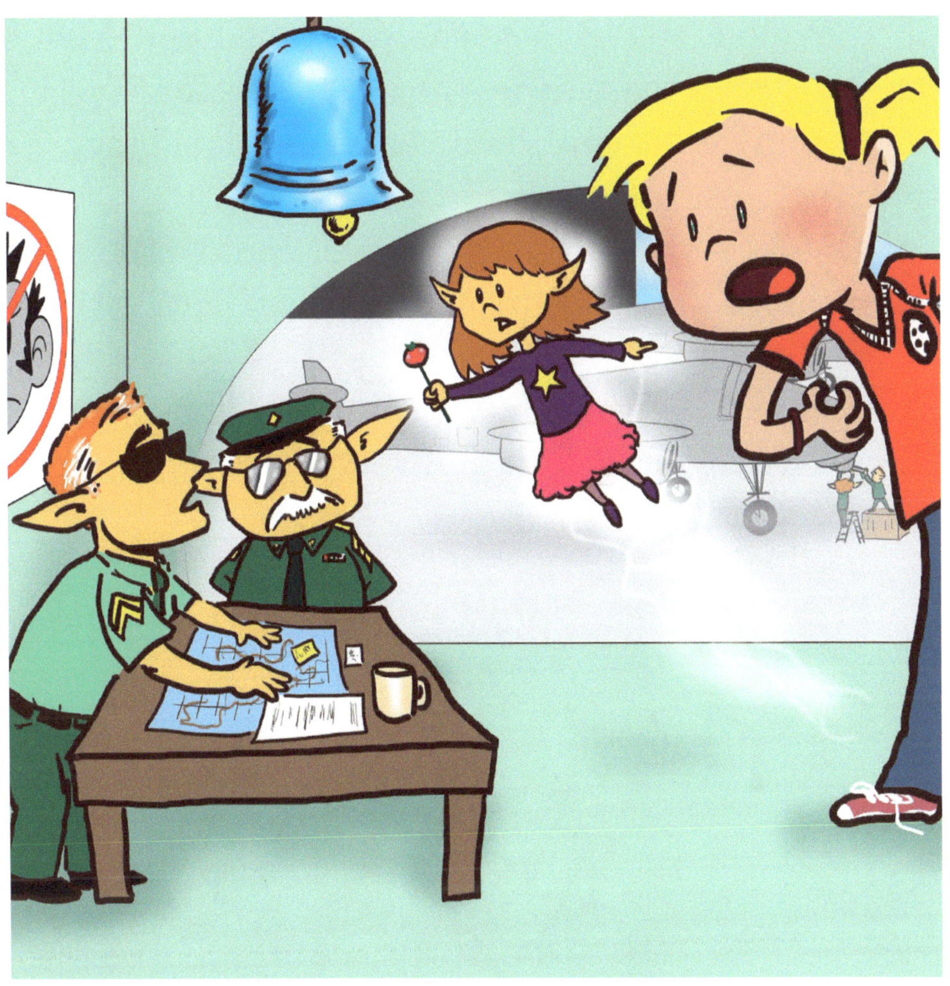

Stargold warned the Elf captain, and he rang a big blue bell to alert the Pilot Elves to get to their planes. As Lucie and Stargold watched, the planes rolled out onto the runway and took off one by one.

"When the Mayhem Monkeys come, they cause damage to our houses!" said Stargold.

"How can we stop them?" Lucie asked.

"Well, Lucie, this is where we need YOU! We need lasers to scare away the Mayhem Monkeys, but we only get them when you eat antioxidants from fruit and vegetables."

"Vegetables?! Ewww!" Lucie shuddered. "Vegetables are sooo gross. But if they turn into lasers, that's pretty cool."

Stargold waved her wand and a tray full of fabulously-coloured fruit and vegetables appeared.

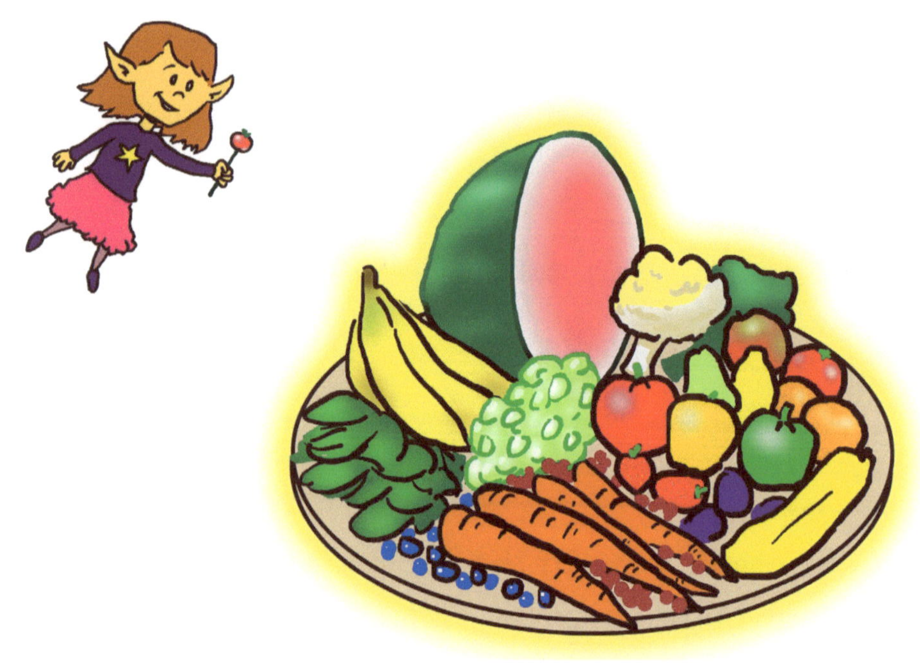

"Now come with me, I will show you!" said Stargold.

They hurried to the runway. Stargold continued: "These boxes are full of lasers. As soon as they arrive, they are loaded onto the planes. Once loaded, the pilots will be equipped to zap the mayhem monkeys."

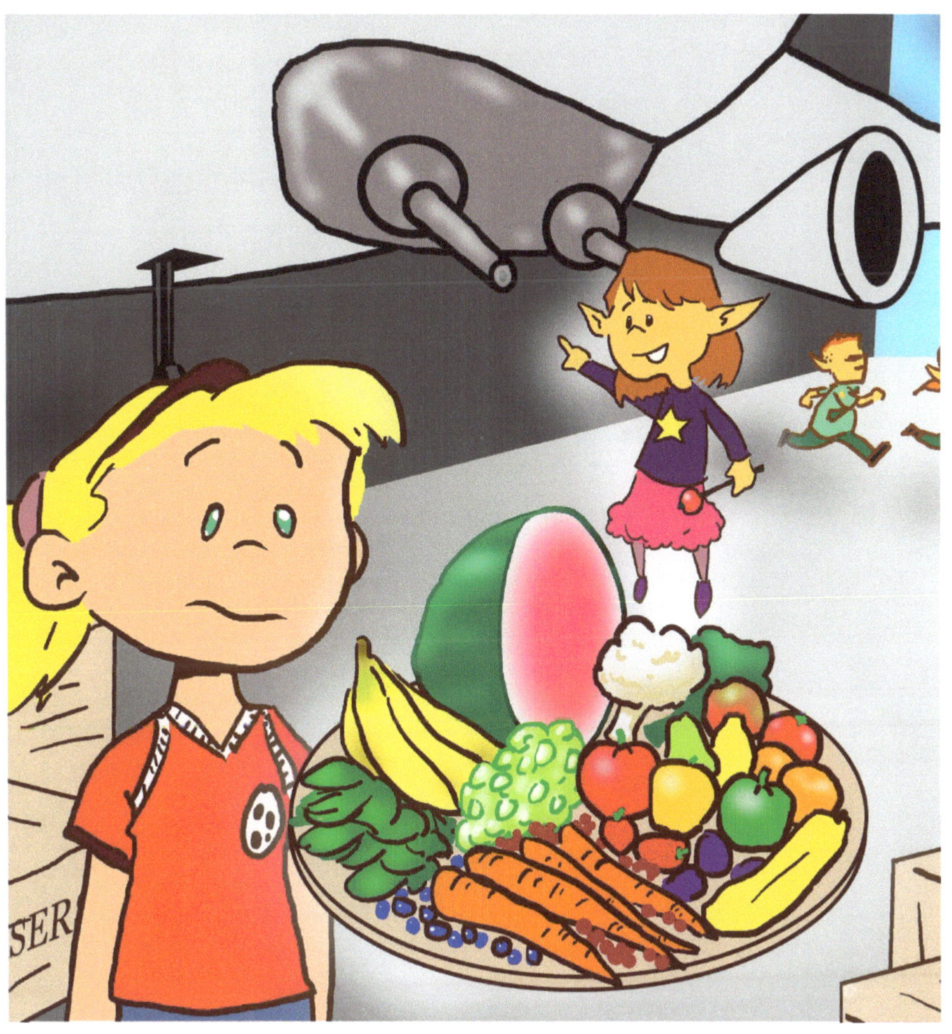

"So eat up, Lucie! The Pilot Elves need lasers!"

Lucie stared at the tray. She made a face at the kale, but grabbed some carrots and broccoli and started eating. It sure didn't taste like candy, but it was crunchy and fresh.

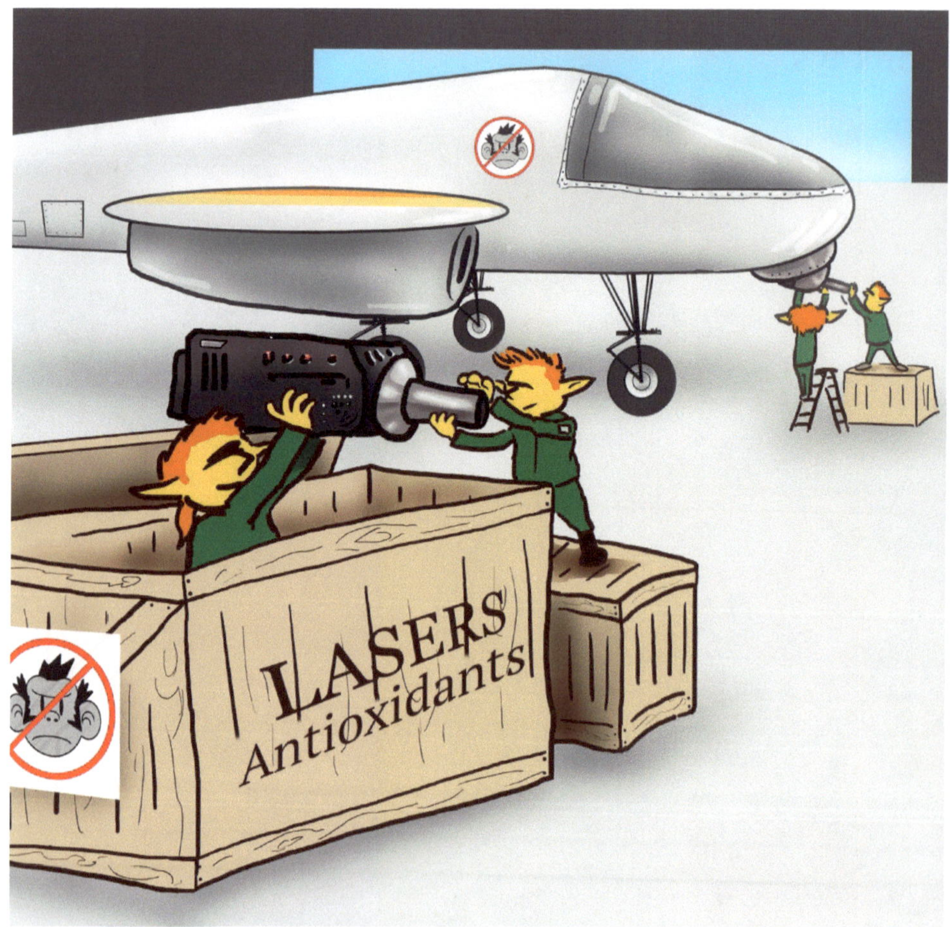

As she chewed, she saw the Rescue Planes pummelling the Mayhem Monkeys with their fabulously-coloured lasers.

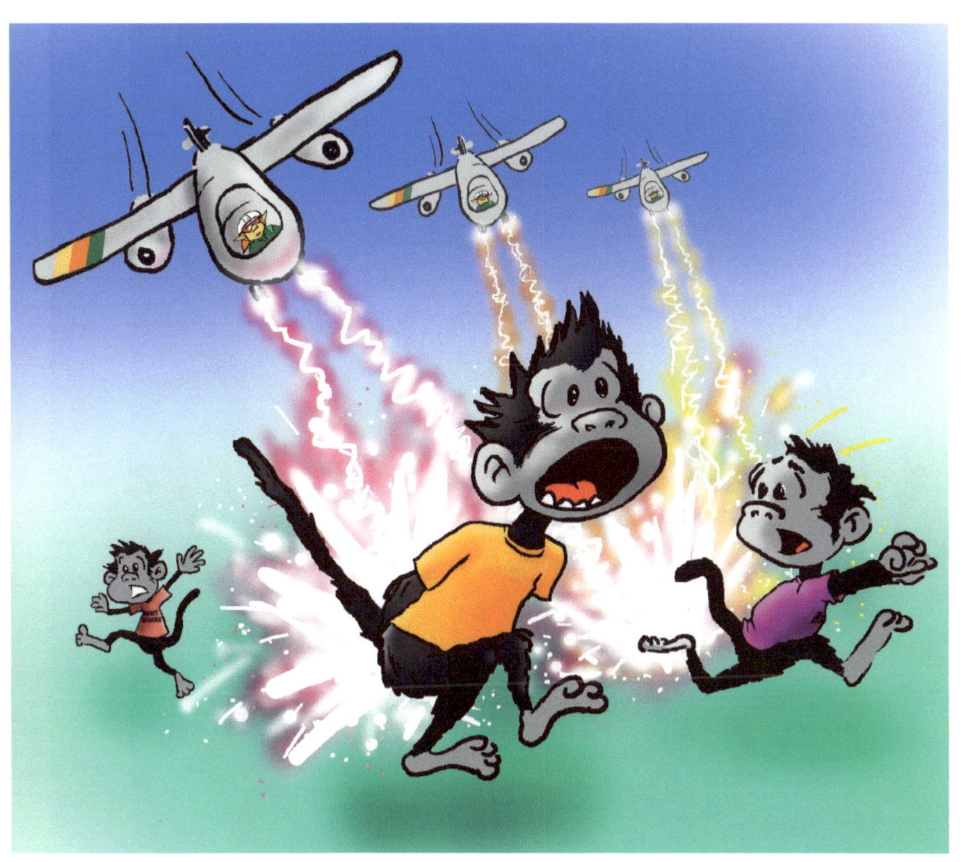

Everyone cheered as the Mayhem Monkeys
ran away.

"Hooray!" yelled Lucie. "We got rid of the monkeys!"

"No, YOU got rid of the monkeys, Lucie" said
Stargold. "When you eat fruits and vegetables, your
body is better at fighting off bad stuff."

"Ooh! That's why Mommy made me that
vegetable and tofu scramble."

"Exactly," said Stargold with a big smile.
Lucie smiled back.

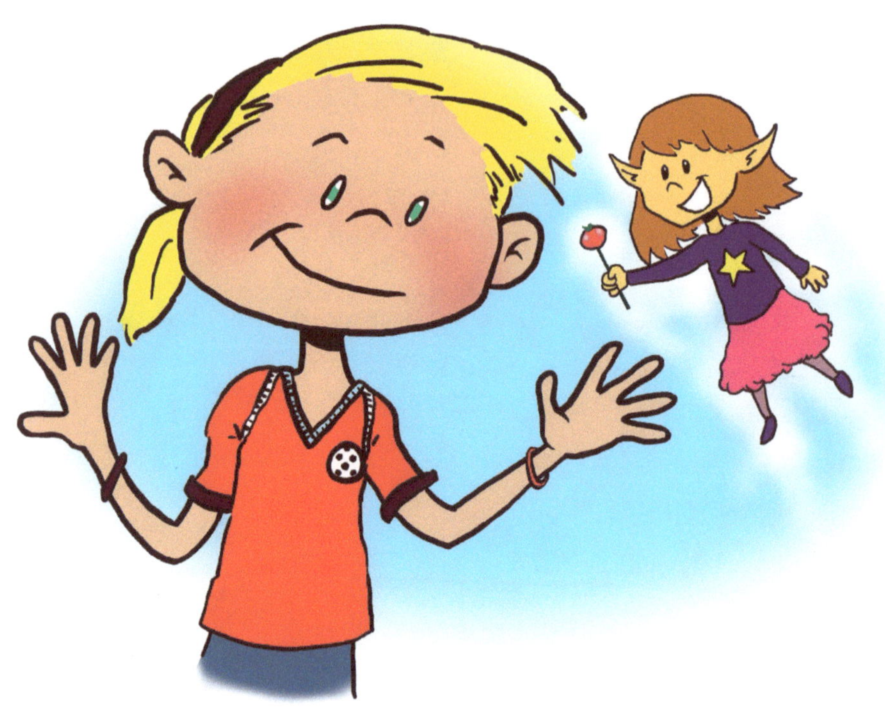

"As you can see," said Stargold, "every last part of your body came from the food you ate. Look at your hands. Look at your feet. Feel your heart beating. These all used to be food!" Lucie stared at her hands in awe.

"Also, listen to your body. It will tell you how much to eat. Treats are fine, as long as you mostly eat the foods that will keep your house strong and healthy."

By then, it was time to go home. Stargold took Lucie's hand and up in the sky they flew.

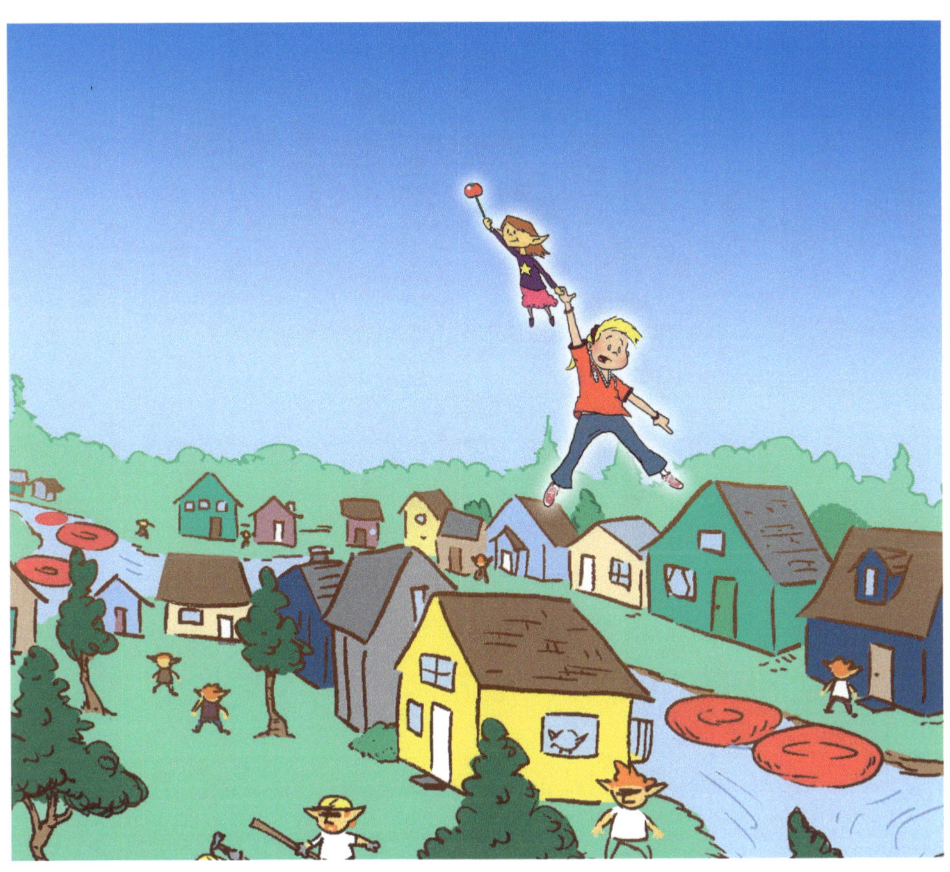

They soared over the giant forest again, flew over the waterfalls, deserts and oceans, to finally arrive back in Lucie's bedroom.

"Thank you so much for showing me Growland," said Lucie. "It was amazing!"

"You are most welcome," said Stargold.

"I will miss you."

"I will miss you too, Lucie," said Stargold.

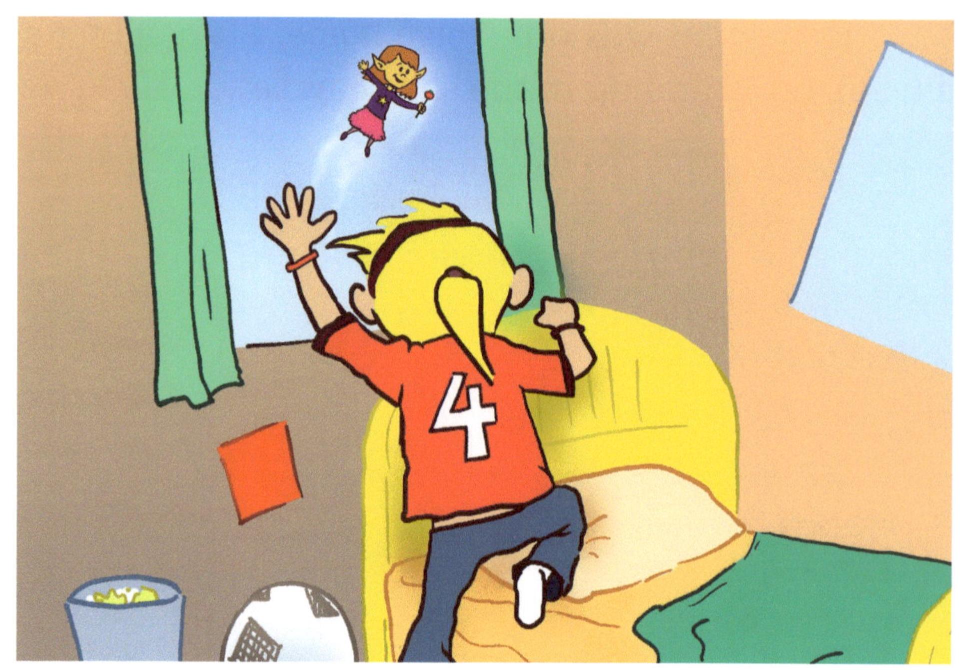

"But we will meet again. In 22 years and 44 days, to be exact, you will need me to talk to your son because he won't eat your veggie pâté."

"No way!" said Lucie. She jumped off her bed and they hugged goodbye. Stargold smiled one last time and left on her rainbow.

Lucie ran back downstairs.

"Mommy, Daddy! I have the most amazing story to tell you! But first, where is that vegetable tofu scramble you made!?"

The End

Lucie's Food Guidance:
To be confident that your child's diet is complete, center his or her diet on the food groups on The Vegan Plate food guide that follows. Pay extra attention to the following nutrients:

Vitamin D
Choose a milk (plant-based) that has been enriched (fortified) with vitamin D. (Read the labels). Children need 15 mcg (600 IU) of Vitamin D daily. Most of these fortified beverages contain about 3.75 mcg (150 IU) per half-cup. It is often advisable to top up vitamin D intake with Vitamin D supplements in the range of 10 mcg (400 IU) per day.

Calcium
Choose plant-based milks or juices that are enriched (fortified) with calcium. Choose tofu that is high in calcium (read the labels). You may top up your child's intake with calcium supplements. Here are recommended daily intakes based on your child's age:

1-3 years old: 700 mg/day
4-8 years old: 1000 mg/day
9-18 years old: 1300 mg/day

Vitamin B12

Vitamin B12 is not present in plant foods. Vitamin B12, including that in animal products and in supplements comes from bacteria. Meet your child's needs for vitamin B12 with one of the following:

-Daily supplement of 10 to 25 mcg
-Twice weekly supplement of 375 mcg
-Vitamin B12 fortified foods (such as non-dairy milk, veggie "meats") two or three times per day

Omega 3 fatty acids
(Alpha-linolenic acid and DHA)

Each day, include 1 tsp chia or hemp seeds or 2 tablespoons of walnuts.
A DHA supplement (in the range of 70 mg DHA/ docosahexaenoic acid) is optional.

Iodine

Daily recommended intakes for iodine can be provided by a multivitamin-mineral supplement (90 mcg iodine for ages 1 to 8, and 120 mcg for ages 9 to 13) Though salt intake should be moderate, iodized salt is also a source (1 ml or 1/5 tsp iodized salt at ages 1 to 8, and 1.5 ml or 1/4 tsp at ages 9 to 18).

THE VEGAN PLATE

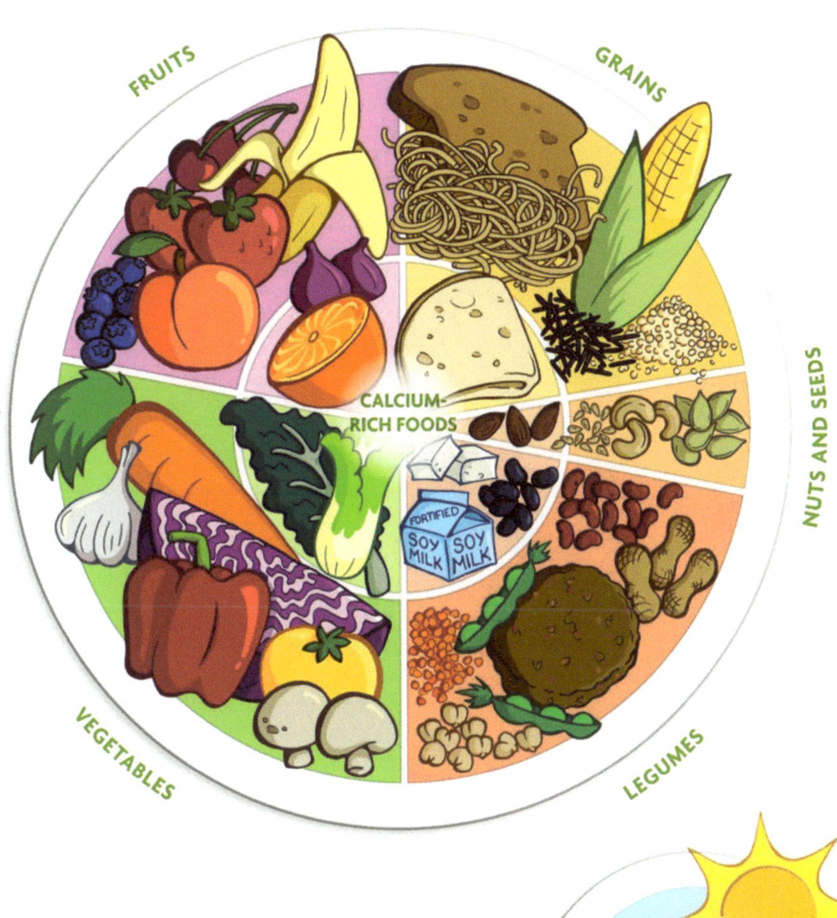

The Vegan Plate food guide from "Becoming Vegan: Comprehensive Edition" and "Becoming Vegan: Express Edition", both by Registered Dietitians Brenda Davis and Vesanto Melina, The Book Publishing Co. (Used with permission)

http://becomingvegan.ca/food-guide/

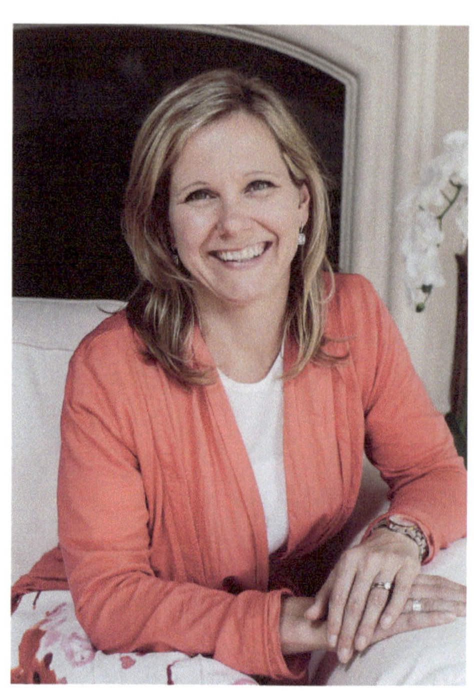

Claudia Lemay, RD
Author

Claudia Lemay resides in Surrey, British Columbia, Canada with her husband, two kids and six pets. She works in a long-term care facility as a clinical dietitian and runs a private practice for picky eaters. She also wrote a sequel to Stargold the Food Fairy called Lucie, Brody and the Food Fairy. This sequel was written to explain diabetes to children.

To learn more about Stargold and healthy nutrition for children, or to find out how to order educational posters or this story in a teacher's presentation version, please visit www.stargoldthefoodfairy.com.

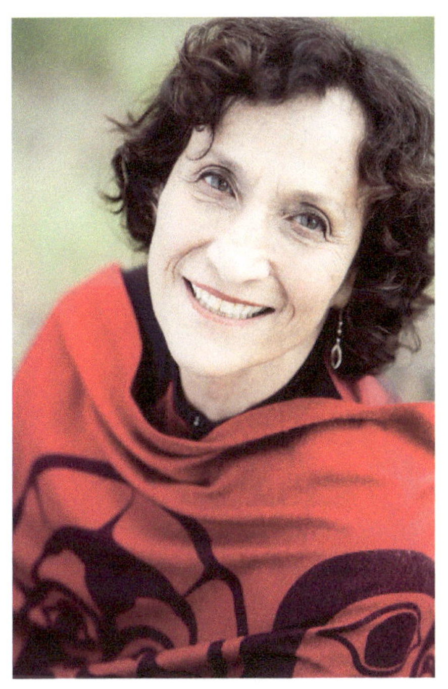

Vesanto Melina, MS, RD
Co-Author

Vesanto Melina, MS, RD is co-author of books that are classics on plant-based nutrition. She co-authored 10 books on plant-based nutrition, now in 11 languages and with 750,000 copies in print. Vesanto has taught nutrition at the University of British Columbia and at Seattle's Bastyr University and is a government consultant. Her speaking engagements with dietetic organizations and other health professionals have taken her across North America and Europe.
Her websites are www.nutrispeak.com and www.becomingvegan.ca

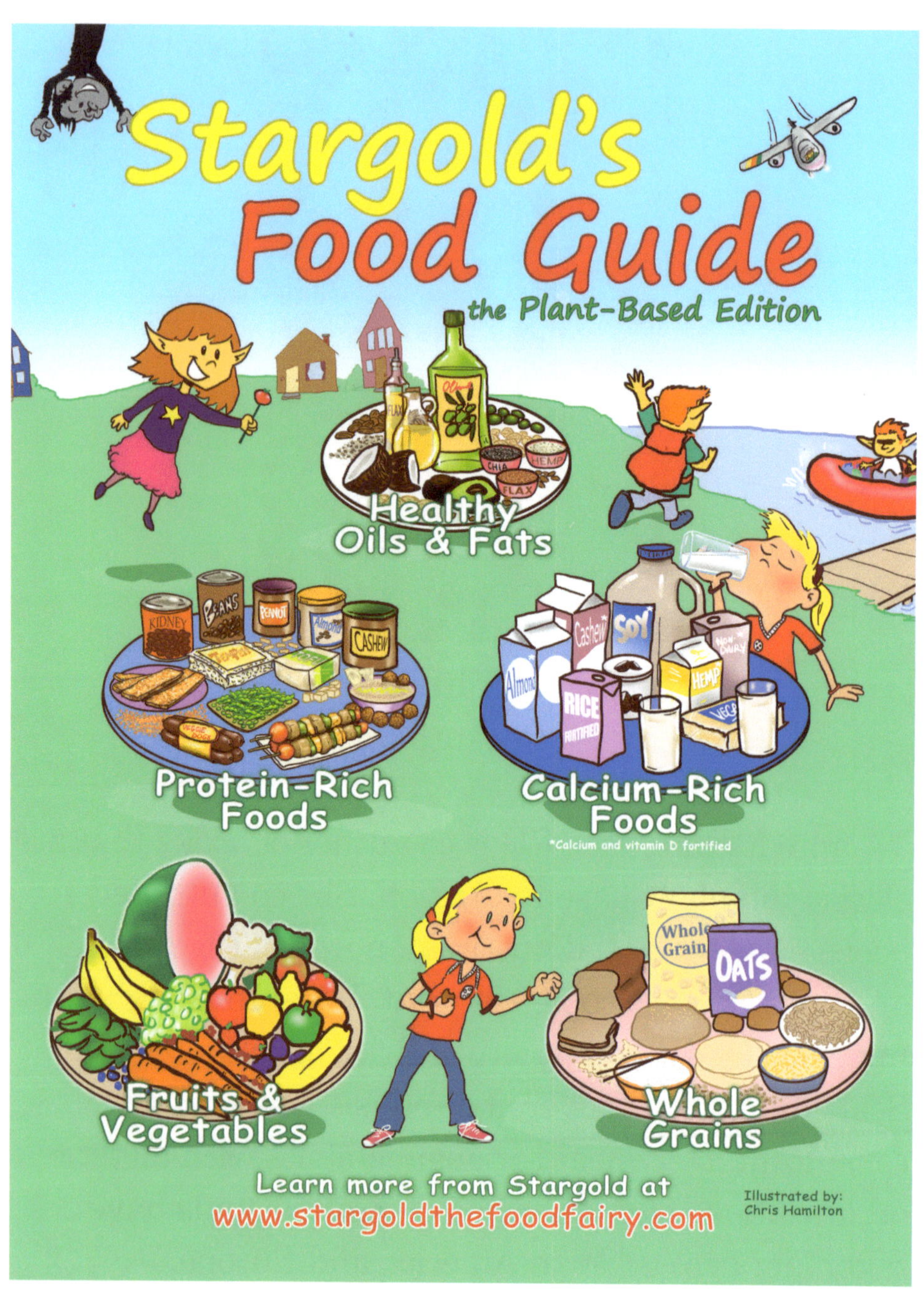

To order copies of "Stargold's Food Guide" in poster format, visit www.stargoldthefoodfairy.com